MW01292341

If It Fits Your Macros

The Ultimate Beginner's Guide

By Jon Peterson

Disclaimer

This book is for informational purposes only. Use of the guidelines in this book is a choice of the reader. This book is not intended for the treatment or prevention of disease. This book is also, not a substitute for medical treatment or an alternative to medical advice.

Table of Contents

Chapter 1

What is If It Fits Your Macros?

IIFYM is a method of dieting used to improve body composition by tracking macronutrients (macros). There are three main macros that are traditionally accounted for: protein, carbs, and fats. By tracking macros, you naturally track your calories as well.

This way of dieting has been gaining vast popularity and chances are you've heard of it. If you've done any research on IIFYM in the past you've, perhaps, realized that no foods are off limits. No food groups are labeled good or bad for you. What matters, in this style of dieting, is if your macro budget has room for the foods you want to eat. If so then you're in the clear, but more on that soon.

So how did this type of dieting come about? Well, bodybuilder's in the old days simply got tired of eating the same bland foods when preparing for a competition. They ate the kind of food that scares people away from attempting to lose weight in the first place! These boring, clean foods, included chicken, broccoli, rice, veggies, eggs, and well—you get the picture. There's no denying that this *bro science* approach to dieting works, but the real question is: is it worth it? After years of making bodybuilders miserable If It Fits Your Macros was born. IIFYM is thus a way to improve one's body composition by not solely relying on clean foods.

A common misconception of IIFYM is that it's just an excuse to eat junk food every day. This is not the case. Contrary to popular belief, IIFYM is not about eating pop tarts for breakfast every day. Unlike traditional diets, you have the *option* to eat what you want, when you want, if you make it fit into your eating plans.

Although the option to eat so-called dirty foods (pizza, burgers, ice cream, cookies etc.) exists, you certainly don't have to part take in it. The edge that IIFYM dieting has over traditional dieting is its flexibility. This flexibility offers you the ability to improve your body composition without having to be perfect or strict with your diet behavior.

There's no reason to be super strict or go on a fad diet. The fad diet approach never last and there seems to be one coming out every other month! Specifically, there's no need for dramatic, and unhealthy, calorie restrictions or any elimination of any particular macronutrient (this includes low-carb approaches). Once you understand the fundamentals of calories and macros you'll have a better understanding of why hardcore and fad diets fall short.

IIFYM offers anyone the opportunity to tailor their diets to their favorite nutritious foods, mixing their favorite treats every day, and still make progress towards their fitness goals.

Is it realistic to say that you're never going to eat ice cream, burgers or pizza again? Are your only carbs going to come from veggies (I can't even stand the thought)? Are you really going to trade all these so-called "dirty foods" out for meals consisting of chicken, brown rice, broccoli and maybe some sweet potatoes if you're lucky? My guess is probably not. That approach to weight loss can cause you to have an all-out binge day in the future. Not only would your diet be strict and boring, but you'll most likely gain back all the "strict diet" weight you lost in the first place.

The best fat loss *strategy*, in my experience, has been **IIFYM**. Another name for this revolutionary way of eating is *Flexible Dieting*. IIFYM has been used for years now. Both people who aim to lose fat or build muscle use it.

Although IIFYM can be used for gaining lean muscle mass, *IIFYM: The Ultimate Beginner's Guide* is tailored towards implementing IIFYM for fat loss. This style of eating is more realistic for people who want to lose fat and enjoy the process.

The benefits of IIFYM:

- Realistic & psychologically beneficial;
- A long-term approach to a healthy lifestyle;
- Compatible with the energy balance law (more on this in Chapter 2);
- Flexible food choices;
- It works perfectly with My Fitness Pal (IIFYM-friendly smartphone app).

This approach, to fat loss, is centered around knowing your macros and hitting your daily macro goals.

My Fitness Pal is the number one tool that makes IIFYM easy to implement.

The following chapters are the fundamentals that you'll need to know in order to integrate IIFYM into your daily routine.

Chapter 2

The Fundamentals of Calories

"Everything is energy and that's all there is to it. Match the frequency of the reality you want and you cannot help but get that reality. It can be no other way. This is not philosophy. This is physics."

— Albert Einstein

Weight loss is derived from universal laws at its core. There's one law in particular that explains how we lose weight. The body obeys the first law of thermodynamics. The first law simply states that energy can neither be created nor destroyed and is often referred to as the energy balance equation (or energy balance law).

$$\Delta U = Q - W$$

(Change in Internal Energy) = (Heat) - (Work)

This law gets the credit for how much weight we lose or gain.

A calorie, by definition, is a unit of heat energy.

If you eat more than your body requires every day, you're bound to gain weight. Gaining weight typically means the body is in a **caloric surplus**. Unwanted fat stores are attributed to the excess intake of these, hopefully, delicious units of energy.

If you eat less than your body needs every day, you're going to lose weight. Losing weight is attributed to being in a **caloric deficit**.

4

Our bodies can also be at equilibrium, meaning our weight remains the same. In this case, the body is at a **caloric maintenance** level.

Does this mean that you can eat whatever you want while in a caloric deficit and still lose weight? Yes, it's possible, but ill-advised. People who try this usually neglect certain macronutrient nourishment, which we'll discuss in more detail later on in this book.

The focus of this book is on losing weight, specifically from fat, while being in a caloric deficit and not in misery at the same time!

When the energy balance equation is applied to fitness, it simply translates to energy (foods) that enters the body and energy that leaves the body as either work (exercise) or heat.

$$\Delta E = E_{in} - E_{out}$$

(Change in Body Weight) = (Energy Consumed) - (Energy Expended)

I'm of the opinion that weight should come off as fast as possible! I don't want to be guessing (eyeballing portions) and hoping I'm in a caloric deficit. I've tried that approach (the eating clean foods approach) to weight loss and I can confirm it's a drag. There's no need to drag out the weight loss process. That approach to weight loss usually leads to people quitting because of a mix of frustration and disappointing progress.

I know one thing for certain: numbers don't lie.

A usual concern for people starting IIFYM is thinking about numbers or math. IIFYM only requires algebra gymnastics if you don't take advantage of IIFYM-friendly apps. Food tracking apps like MyFitnessPal (MFP) have been created to make tracking food consumption a breeze. MFP does all the heavy lifting (the math) for you! Here's an example:

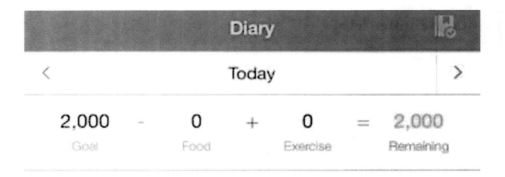

Look familiar? It's the energy balance equation in action slightly rearranged.

The easiest way to start IIFYM is by logging in what you eat with MFP. If you choose to you can track your exercise as well!

We'll be using MFP as our food tracker because it's the most highly rated and popular food tracking app available. Think of this app as the fuel gauge in your car. You wouldn't want to go on a road trip from California to Washington with your fuel gauge broken. You might make it to your destination, but you will encounter a variety of unnecessary obstacles along the way.

Knowing how much fuel is in the "tank" is imperative to losing weight in a timely manner. MFP will be your energy fuel gauge. This handy app will give you an insight into why you're getting closer or further to your goal. Knowing your total calorie consumption carries the potential to save you time on your journey. In other words, it eliminates guessing and if you value time like I do then guessing is something you do not want to be associated with.

MFP can be used on any smart device (iPhone, Android, iPad/tablet, or on a regular computer). Most people use their smartphones to track their food intake because it's the most convenient option, namely because your phone's camera can be a barcode scanner.

I'll be showing you step-by-step examples on how to track your food, and thus your macros, on an iPhone (MFP's user interface is similar and consistent across all smart devices). Before we get started, it's time for you to take your first action step!

Action Step 1
Download MFP, an IIFYM-friendly app, onto your smart device.

Chapter 3

Getting Started with MFP

3.1 How to Set Up Your Daily Caloric Goal with MFP

When it comes to healthy weight loss, the rule of thumb is to lose 1 to 2 pounds per week for both men and women. Weight loss slowly decreases as the weeks go on and progress is achieved. It's not uncommon to only lose 0.5 to 1 pound per week when you're trying to lose those last few pounds of stubborn belly fat!

For overweight individuals, it's common to lose more than 10 pounds in the first month of being in a caloric deficit. The more weight you have to lose initially, the greater amount of weight that'll come off. Be aware that this initial weight won't entirely be from fat stores. A good portion of that weight will be water weight. Nevertheless, this is still a great sign and a step in the right direction.

By now you should have MFP on your smartphone. Let's get started.

Step 1: Select a Goal

For the Goal selection, select *Lose Weight*.

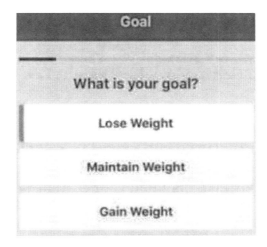

Step 2: Select Activity Level

Keep in mind that this question doesn't take exercising into consideration. If you feel like changing the activity level for your account, you can do so in *settings* at any time.

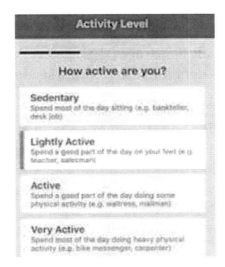

Step 3 & 4: Basic Information

These two steps are titled "You" and are self-explanatory steps that include basic information on age and body measurements.

Step 5: Setting Weekly Weight Loss Goals

I encourage you to start off at 1 pound per week for this step. I found with a selection of more than 1 pound per week, MFP will assume you're ready to go into a very low-calorie deficit and will shave off 1,000+ calories from your maintenance calories (the number of calories to maintain your current weight) in some cases.

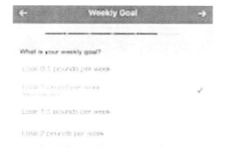

Don't have analysis paralysis! You can change your caloric deficit in the *settings* section.

3.2 Adjusting Initial Calories

If you're unsatisfied with the calories MFP gives you (not uncommon) then I encourage you to find a caloric deficit that works best for you. There are multiple methods to get your caloric deficit numbers, but one of the easiest ways I found was using an online flexible dieting calculator (healthyeater.com/flexible-dieting-calculator).

This resource will give you a great estimate for your caloric deficit. A quick note on calorie intake: Every method you use will be an estimate.

Here's how you would change the default calories MFP assigns:

1. Select "More"

2. Select "Goals" then -> "Nutrition Goals"

3. Select "Calories" and enter your appropriate calories.

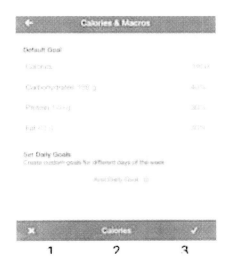

You're now signed up and ready to use MFP. Next, let's discuss how to log in foods using MFP.

3.3 *How to Log in Foods*
There are two methods of logging in food:

1) Searching MFP's food directory

2) Barcode scanning

When you're on the diary screen select +*Add Food* to use either method. Once you've selected that the following screen, below, will appear and you can use either method.

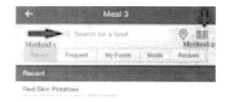

You can use a combination of the two methods or use them individually. For example, I was able to scan this delicious treat (dark chocolate) into my food diary using my phone's camera.

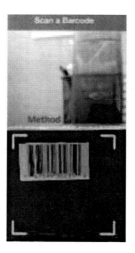

In my experience, barcode scanning works most of the time. The majority of grocery barcodes reveal a lot of nutritional information via MFP. When barcodes are scanned, MFP will display the nutrition facts of the food product along with its standard serving size on your smart device. What makes MFP powerful is that you can adjust your serving sizes!

On rare occasions, when a certain food doesn't have a barcode, use Method 1 to log in the food entry.

There are times when Method 1 is better suited than Method 2. This is common when you log in produce foods. Foods such as apples or bananas usually don't come with barcodes (unless you buy them in a bulk bag).

Method 1 is essentially using MFP's extensive food database. For example, when I log in apples, I type in "Red apple generic" and a list of options become available. I pick the most appropriate selection and I'm set. Method 1 will also be ideal when we discuss IIFYM and eating out in chapter 5.

In either method, keep in mind that MFP will provide you with the default nutrition label serving size.

3.4 Measuring Food Servings

"What gets measured, gets managed." – Peter Drucker

Weight loss is a numbers game, not a guessing game. When it comes to certain foods, having measuring tools for volume and weight can be very helpful. These tools are meant to eliminate guessing and to ensure we're in a caloric deficit every day until we've reached our weight loss goal.

For example, it's easy to overestimate (or underestimate) a tablespoon of olive oil. One tablespoon of olive oil is roughly 120 calories and eyeballing an olive oil serving, even as little as ½ a tablespoon a day, can add up! If people were to reflect on how much oils, sauces, treats, or dressings they use in their cooking, it could potentially be an eye opener. This quick evaluation can be a game changer in some people's weight loss journeys.

Meats can also vary in thickness which factors into the overall serving size. I don't know about you, but I don't feel comfortable eyeballing 8 ounces of steak or a 2/3 cup serving of mashed potatoes. I assume I'm not in the minority here. Enter kitchen measuring tools.

Here's a list of measuring tools that I recommend for IIFYM with MFP:

- Kitchen food scale (oz./grams)

- Measuring Cup(s)

- Measuring Spoon Set

Use these measuring tools when you log in foods that require it. There are some foods that don't need to be measured too seriously. Let me explain. If you purchase a bag of apples and the nutrition label states that each apple is *about 5.5 oz.*, then there's really no need to weigh each apple out and test it. You'll be fine logging 5.5 ounces into MFP.

It's funny, when I first started using MFP for IIFYM, I would obsess and weigh each apple on my kitchen food scale. The difference was so minuscule that I'd shave off one measly calorie, and if I was lucky maybe two!

Also, don't worry about having to re-enter your meals every day; MFP has got you covered with a cool feature which we'll discuss very soon.

3.5 Tracking Exercise

MFP gives you the option to add exercise to your energy balance equation. I say, option, because it's not 100% necessary if you're already following a sound fitness program.

There are two categories of exercise that MFP offers. The first being Cardio and second Strength Training (a.k.a. weight lifting). Both vitally important to body composition in their own right.

Logging in cardio is a good idea if your exercise is solely coming from cardiorespiratory activity. It's definitely a good idea if you're new to tracking your food intake because MFP shows you how exercise affects your energy balance equation. You'll notice you have more calories burned, in the equation display screen, after logging your cardio exercise.

The process of tracking your calories burned is simple.

First, a quick note on cardio machines: When you step onto the cardio machine of your choice, make sure to input your age, weight and anything else the cardio machine requests. Most people skip this step and usually jump right into their workout by pressing the "Quick start" button.

The reason you want to input your information is to get the most accurate reading possible for your workout. In other words, you want to know how many calories you burned during your workout as accurately as possible.

Once your cardio workout is complete, record the number of calories burned displayed on your cardio machine's screen, post workout, and log it into MFP.

Unfortunately, logging Strength Training in MFP doesn't adjust your energy balance equation. MFP allows you to log in a list of your strength training workouts, but nothing more. This is because there currently are no devices that track your energy expenditure while strength training. Strength training involves many variables which makes it hard to measure a set number of calories burned for a particular lifting session. Such variables include:

- Varying weights used throughout a workout;

- Amount of sets, repetitions, and the rest time in between those sets;

- The intensity of weight lifting which varies in each individual.

Although you can lose weight from being in a caloric deficit alone, there is a better strategy. If you combine a caloric deficit with cardiovascular *and* strength training, you will accelerate your weight loss effort.

I recommend a minimum of three days a week for weight training, in combination, with your cardio workouts in order to avoid a non-toned (skinny fat) look. The look most people are after is the strong and lean look at, or around, 10% body fat for men and the toned look at, or around 16% body fat for women. Whichever approach you take, recall that in order to lose weight, it's calories in versus calories out.

Alright, we've now covered the basics of using MFP. It's time to learn more about macros and their role in improving body composition.

Action Step 2

1. Log in a meal you recently ate or are about to eat using MFP.

2. Log in a days' worth of eating using MFP.

Note: If you don't have a food scale, get one at your local store, or online store, as soon as possible. This action step is to practice using the two methods discussed earlier on in this chapter.

The time of guessing your way to your fitness goals is over.

Chapter 4

Macronutrients and Body Composition

"You should measure things you care about. If you're not measuring, you don't care and you don't know" – Steve Howard

4.1 What Are Macros?

Nutrition Facts

Serving Size 1 cup (228g)
Servings Per Container 2

Amount Per Serving

Calories 250	Calories from Fat 110

	% Daily Value*
Total Fat 12g	18%
Saturated Fat 3g	15%
Trans Fat 1.5g	
Cholesterol 30mg	10%
Sodium 470mg	20%
Total Carbohydrate 31g	10%
Dietary Fiber 0g	0%
Sugars 5g	
Protein 5g	

Macronutrients are important when it comes to body composition, diet satiety and adherence. Macronutrients, scientifically, involve the second law of thermodynamics and deals with entropy. The second law states, it's impossible for a system to consume energy and have an equivalent amount of work as a result. A fascinating subject, but the depth in relation to fat loss far exceeds the scope of this book.

To put it simply, the second law states, for body composition, that a calorie is not a calorie. Different macronutrients (proteins, carbohydrates, and dietary fats) have different thermic effects on the body. When you eat foods, the body requires different amounts of energy, depending on the macronutrient, to break it down. It costs energy to digest, absorb and to store those nutrients. Thus, not all calories are created equal.

Macros usually tend to be ignored, not on purpose, but because of a tunnel vision approach to the energy balance law. There's an overemphasis on calorie consumption and not enough on macro consumption, which plays a role on your body's composition. Neglecting a macronutrient intake, from protein, for instance, can lead to losing weight from muscle instead of fat stores. As a result your metabolism will deteriorate over time, which is not the ideal case anyone should be striving for.

In this chapter, you'll discover how the number of calories you consume are proportionally related to your macros.

Keeping track of macronutrients, specifically, the percentage that each macronutrient contributes towards your daily caloric goal makes your fat loss journey far more enjoyable. Knowing how much protein, carbohydrates, and fat to eat every day will help you stay full and satisfied. Feeling full is incredibly important when you're in a caloric deficit. Despite what you may have heard, being in a caloric deficit is not supposed to be a miserable experience or a test of your willpower!

Before proceeding, on how MFP handles macros and macro recommendations, let's briefly cover some fundamentals of macronutrients in the nutrition realm. This will make sense of how macronutrients are related to calories.

Although there's some minor math involved in this next section, don't worry! Once again, MFP can handle all these calculations for you. Afterward, I'll show you exactly how to account for macros using MFP.

4.2 Macros 101
The following section is to provide you with a solid foundation as to *why* macronutrients are important to your body and fat loss journey. MFP tracks macros in grams.

Protein

(1 gram of protein = 4 calories)

The building blocks of proteins are amino acids. Amino acids are responsible for repairing and building muscle tissue. There two types of amino acids: essential and nonessential amino acids. The body can manufacture the nonessential amino acids and relies on you to feed it the essential amino acids which come in the form of protein.

Protein tends to be the most commonly neglected macronutrient and usually takes a backseat behind carbs and fats. There are, however, good reasons not to neglect protein.

First, protein-rich foods provide satiety, which is essential to feeling full when you're a few hundred calories below maintenance. Studies show that humans preloaded with protein have their food intake suppressed for several hours.

Second, protein has the greatest thermic effect out of the three macros. Meaning, eating protein takes more energy (calories) to digest, absorb, and store than carbs or fats. You're actually burning more calories when you eat protein.

Here's a list of some major quality protein sources:

- Meat and poultry;

- Fish (salmon, tuna, tilapia etc.);

- Dairy Products (milk, cottage cheese etc.);

- Whole eggs & egg whites.

These quality proteins will ensure you're getting your essential amino acids replenished and should be eaten on a regular basis.

Carbohydrates

(1 gram = 4 calories)

Carbs provide the body with the fuel needed for everyday living and help you feel energized throughout the day. They are the essential, must have, fuel source for every cell in the body. This macro is especially vital for fitness enthusiasts and maximal sports performance.

Carbs also aid in the digestion and utilization of proteins and fat. The body prefers carbs for energy because it's the one macronutrient that is most efficiently turned into energy for the body to use.

There's no need to go on a low, or zero, carb diet when your goal is fat loss. I've lost weight without going low on carbs. Low carb diets are unrealistic for long-term success. Low carb has been made popular through media such as fitness magazines, and people in the mainstream media. They promise fast weight loss, but the majority of that weight is water weight and at times, muscle glycogen. Sure the scale goes down, but now you have the skinny fat look and you're prone to regain the weight you lost.

I fell into the low carb trap once. This approach made my journey miserable, I felt sluggish, and wasn't satisfied with the process at the end of the day. Anytime you find yourself feeling miserable in the weight loss process that's a sign that there are adjustments needed to be made.

When I reintroduced carbs into my diet, I felt full and satisfied again. Everything became easier and the weight still kept coming off. Carbs are your friend and contrary to popular belief, not evil!

There are two types of carbohydrates: complex carbs and simple carbs. Complex carbs come from complex starches such as those found in whole grains and vegetables. I find complex carbs such as beans, sweet potatoes, and wheat bread to be the most satiating. Simple carbs are foods such as white potatoes and white rice. I like having a good balance between the two types of carbs, but everyone is different.

At the end of the day both, types of carbs, get converted into glucose (a.k.a. blood sugar) in the body. Keep it simple, remember that as long as you're in a caloric deficit, you'll continue to lose weight. White carbs are not to blame for your inability to lose fat, that usually boils down to the energy balance law.

Pick carbs that you enjoy eating, and never fear carbs as they're necessary for fueling your body throughout your weight loss process.

Here's a list of carbohydrates that I found nutritiously dense and filling:

- Potatoes

- Sweet Potatoes

- Lentils

- White/brown rice

- Fruits

- Vegetables

- Bread

- Yogurt

- Rice Cakes

Dietary Fat

(1 gram of fat = 9 calories)

This last macro has more than twice as many calories per gram as protein and carbohydrates.

Fats have also gotten a bad rap over the years; back in the 90's, dietary fat was vilified of being "bad for you" especially if your goal was to lose fat.

That myth has been debunked over the last decades, but one thing was true. Dietary fats (the kind you eat) are the one macronutrient that's most easily converted into body fat. An excess of dietary fats, in our diets, lead to additional body fat stores. According to Robert E. T. Stark, MD, who was the past president of the American Society of Bariatric Physicians, more than 90% of dietary calories we consume end up as body fat stores.

The trick is to get the right type of fats and the adequate amount of it in our diets. We should be consuming dietary fats that promote hormone balance, supplement the fat loss process, and contribute energy. The good news is that dietary fat provides flavor and promotes satiety.

I'll break it down into two camps; good fats, and bad fats. Dietary fats are made up of fatty acids.

Good fats consist of essential fatty acids (EFA) needed by the human body. These EFA's provide the body with energy, hormone regulation, digestion.

The body can't survive without EFAs and therefore, we get them from healthy food sources.

Here's a list of good fats:

- Olive oil

- Coconut oil

- Avocados

- Peanuts

- Almonds

- Salmon

Of course, with the good comes some bad. The bad fats are man-made and are called trans-fats. Trans-fats can be found in foods such as ice cream, cookies, cereals, fried foods and lots of processed foods.

Trans-fatty acids are responsible for raising the bad kind of cholesterol: LDL (low-density lipoproteins). Other side effects include heart disease, type 2 diabetes, and clog up arteries.

My experience with trans-fat has been that they're not filling at all. For example, I love Circus Animal Cookies, I would keep them in my kitchen pantry except I would cheat too often.

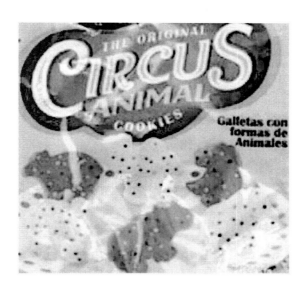

Honestly, I used to sneak them in without logging them into MFP! Let me tell you, those added up quickly with or without tracking macros!

Even when I did log these cookies in MFP, I found myself feeling hungry throughout the day. Keep in mind that I was still in a caloric deficit when I logged these cookies in. I had to remove the temptations of these types of snacks in order not to plateau during my weight loss journey. If you can handle these being around the kitchen, and they fit your macros, go for it! My self-control abilities go out the window when I'm around cookies.

Back to trans-fats. Food companies try their best to hide trans-fats in the nutrition labels, thus being nutrition literate is important. Take a look at the following Circus Animal cookies nutrition label:

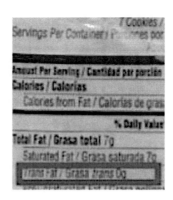

They claim to have zero trans fats in their cookies. Am I lying to you then? Not really, they actually do have trans-fat in them, but FDA regulations state if the amount is less than ½ a gram of trans-fat in a food serving then the food manufacturer can label the product as zero grams of trans-fat. I don't know about you, but I can't stop at one serving of these cookies!

Beware of the ingredients list. The list won't specifically tell you that trans-fats are included. No, that'd be far too easy. Trans-fats will be cloaked by words that start with *hydrogenated*.

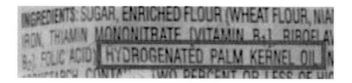

Foods that often contain trans-fats are:

- Tortilla chips

- Cakes, cookies, & pastries

- Deep fried foods (French fries and doughnuts come to mind).

Never having these foods again, quitting cold turkey, is unrealistic. Moderation is the key when eating foods that come from the "bad fats" camp.

4.3 Macronutrient Recommendations

The format in which I'll be addressing macros are as follows:

Protein / Carbs / Fat.

This type of format is often called "macro splits" or "macro ratios". It's a form of distributing your macros amongst your daily caloric intake by percentages.

Macronutrient recommendations, according to the Institutes of Medicine, calculated the following acceptable ranges:

- 10-35% of calories should come from protein;

- 45-65% of calories should come from carbohydrates;

- 20-35% of calories should come from fats.

Although these ranges are good, they're quite broad and not specific enough for someone who is aiming to lose body fat and have a good body composition.

The following macro ratios are common, amongst the IIFYM community, and I've also used them myself with great success:

1. 40/40/20

2. 30/40/30

3. 30/45/25

Note: You can use any of the above three ratios and lose weight. As long as you remain in a caloric deficit (obeying the law of energy balance) these ratios should work for most people beginning IIFYM.

Let's put macro ratios into perspective by using the third ratio option.

We'll use a 200 lb. male for our example and use the **30/45/25** ratio.

Caloric Deficit (20% deficit) = 2,400 calories

30% of calories from protein = 0.30 x 2,400 = 720 calories

Grams of protein per day = 720 calories ÷ 4 $\frac{grams}{calories}$ = **180 grams of protein per day**

45% of calories from carbs = .45 x 2,400 = 1,080 calories

Grams of carbs per day = 1,080 calories ÷ 4 $\frac{grams}{calories}$ = **270 grams of carbs per day**

25% of calories from dietary fat = .25 x 2,400 = 600 calories

Grams of fat per day = 600 calories ÷ 9 $\frac{grams}{calories}$ = **67 grams of fat per day**

Will you have to do this math? No, because MFP does it for you.

All you have to do is choose the macronutrient ratio that best suits you.

Your macro ratios, just like your caloric intake, are not set in stone.

In the image below, my goal macro ratio is set to 30 (P)/ 40 (C)/ 30 (F) but, on March 23rd, I felt like my body needed more carbs so I didn't follow my macro ratio to the T.

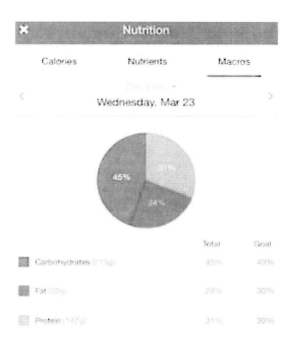

	Total	Goal
Carbohydrates (213g)	45%	40%
Fat (52g)	24%	30%
Protein (147g)	31%	30%

In my experience, protein is the most important macro to hit every day to preserve lean muscle tissue while losing fat. Your carbs and fats are debatable, but I like to keep my carbs relatively high and my fat no lower than 20-25%. To ensure you're not gaining fat, make sure to stay within your daily calorie limit and you're golden; the weight will continue to come off.

Macros play an important role in satiety and your adherence to any fat loss program. They all contain energy and nutrients your body needs. Eating too much of any of them will ultimately contribute to weight gain.

Let's find out how to set up your macronutrient percentages on MFP.

4.4 *Adjusting Your Macronutrient Ratios on MFP*

Setting up your macronutrient ratio is similar to adjusting your caloric intake.

Step 1: Select *More*

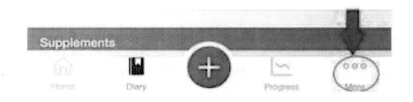

Step 2: Select *Goals*

Step 3: Under *Nutrition Goals* select *Calorie & Macronutrient Goals*

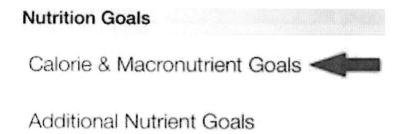

Step 4: Select any of the three listed macronutrients

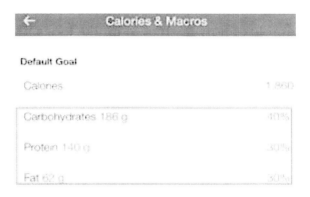

Step 5: Choose a macronutrient ratio that will work best for you.

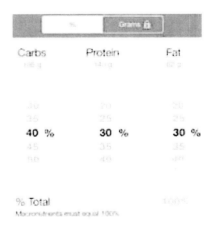

Once complete, MFP will distribute your calories into daily macro targets (in grams) you need to be in your caloric deficit. You can always adjust your calories and macronutrients when you wish.

Don't be afraid to experiment with different macro ratios. Fat loss journeys, are also about learning how your body responds to diet tweaks.

Here's an example of how my macro intake looks like tomorrow. My caloric deficit is 1,860 calories.

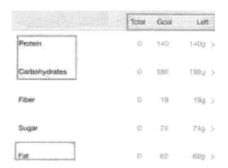

My macro targets are:

- Protein: 140 grams

- Carbs: 186 grams

- Fat: 62 grams

Note: You can get to the above screen by simply tapping on the energy balance equation on the Diary screen.

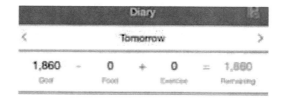

Action Step 3

Choose a macronutrient ratio on MFP, following the steps outlined in this chapter, and try it out for a few days. If you're not satisfied, change it until you find the ratio that's right for you.

Chapter 5

MFP Features for IIFYM Success

"You'll never change your life until you change something you do daily. The secret of your success is found in your daily routine." – John C. Maxwell

At the end of the day it's the people who regulate their food intake who have the greatest successes in their fat loss journeys. I don't even consider logging in food a hassle anymore. Once you start seeing success with IIFYM, the once upon a time "hassle", gets transmuted into a habit.

The price of doing what everyone else does is simple: little to no weight loss progress and a return to old habits. Of course, it's easier to just grab some healthy food and cook it, or in some cases, heating up leftovers. This is the approach most people take.

I want you to have long-term success and in order to do that, in fitness or any other area of life, it requires obtaining new habits. While reading this chapter, remember that you're learning a process that'll take you to your end goal if you make the commitment.

5.1 Saving Time with Meal Entries

When I first started tracking my food I didn't want to think about numbers every time I was going to eat. What I realized was that measuring foods (in ounces, grams, cups, tablespoons etc.) wasn't as bad when you created a meal plan which was tailored just for you, a topic that's coming up soon. Combine a meal plan, with MFP's logging features, and tracking becomes extremely easy.

MFP makes tracking what you eat easy because it upkeeps a history database, similar to an internet browsing history, of the foods you've eaten in the past. Having a database, built into MFP, is great because it easily retrieves past food entries and allows it to be easily added to any meal you choose.

A great shortcut on MFP is the *Smart Copy* feature which has the potential to remove any hassle from food tracking. The *Smart Copy* feature will save you the most time if you have a meal plan, or consistently eat the same meals every day. It quickly lets you add what you ate yesterday (or X amount of days before) to the present day's corresponding meal. You do this with one quick swipe of a finger.

Take the following steps to enable the *Smart Copy* feature. The steps should also be a great example of how this process looks like.

Step 1: Select ••• *More*

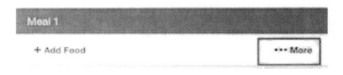

Step 2: Select Turn On Smart Copy

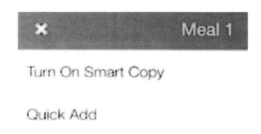

Step 3: Swipe right to add

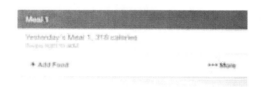

It's as simple as that. You can enable, or disable, this feature for any meal you'd like. Depending on your meal situation, you might need to adjust what gets copied. Sometimes you might want to add or remove a certain food that gets copied from the day before. You're able to approve what gets copied and what doesn't.

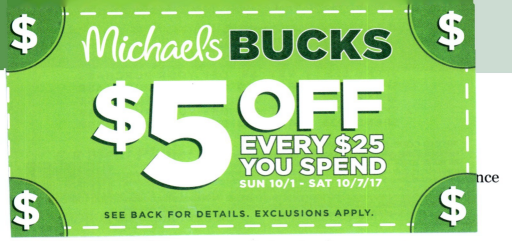

Consider it a better approach than having to consistently ask yourself "Okay... what am I going to eat today?" every few hours of every day. Take the time to create a meal plan and liberate yourself from such decisions.

Take a look at a meal plan I created for myself:

Meal 1:

- Chicken breast (~8-9 oz. uncooked weight)
- Red potatoes (~ 15-16 oz.)
- 2 whole eggs
- 85 grams of broccoli (weighed frozen)
- Light Butter (14 grams)
- Dark Chocolate (1-2 Squares)

Meal 2:

- Chicken Breast (~8-9 oz. uncooked weight)
- Lentil Beans (1 cup)
- Brown Rice (1 cup)
- 1 egg
- 85 grams of broccoli (weighed frozen)
- Light Butter (7 grams)

Meal 3:

- Low Fat Cottage Cheese (1/2 cup)

- Whey Protein (1 scoop)

- Peanut Butter (4 grams)

- Quaker Oats (10 grams)

- Banana (40 grams sliced)

- Stevia Packet

- Walden Farm Zero Calorie Chocolate Syrup

As you can see, I only eat three meals a day and skip breakfast. This is an intermittent fasting example of meal planning, but a meal plan nonetheless. By the way IIFYM and Intermittent fasting complement each other handsomely, but that a topic for a future book.

The great thing about meal plans is that you can tailor them to your needs. Whether that's three, four, five, or six meals a day! Your pick of foods is up for grabs as long as you hit your daily macros. Be strategic on the foods you pick. Make sure to include nutritiously dense foods in each of your meals to ensure satiety. Although you can fit treats into your daily macro limit, be aware that you'll most likely not feel full if they're heavily spread throughout your meal plan. I recommend having your daily treat alongside one of your meals.

An easy way to a create a meal plan is to brainstorm the foods you like to eat and distribute them amongst the amount of meals you'd like to eat every day. You can use grocery items you already have at home and cross check the nutritional values (macros). Simply scan or search foods in MFP and create a meal plan that fits your macros. Creating a meal plan takes time, so set aside some time to complete this task. I usually start this process by writing down my plan and then transferring the final meal plan into a nice spreadsheet.

5.3 Eating Out (Nutrition Info. Available)

Just because you set a fitness goal to improve your health and lifestyle doesn't mean you have to eliminate eating out. Such a tradeoff would be absurd. On days I know I'm going out to eat, I like to plan ahead.

MFP has an awesome feature called, *Create a New Food* under *My Recipes & Foods* in the main menu.

You can take advantage of using this feature by doing some quick Google research on the place you're going to be dining at. The *Create a New Food* feature allows to you input the calories (and macros) you find from your Google research. This easy process involves Googling nutrition information and configuring what you find in your MFP diary.

Unless you want to ask for nutrition information at the restaurant then I suggest you do some quick research before going out to eat (for simplicity, I'll be using the word *restaurant* to describe traditional restaurants and fast food places alike).

Do you have a restaurant in mind?

Good, take a look at the example below. It's an example of me creating a new meal entry, in MFP, for a Chipotle Mexican Grill meal:

Step 1: Google: *"restaurant"* + *nutrition*

Step 2: Select the nutrition calculator option if available

Nutrition Calculator - Chipotle
https://www.chipotle.com/nutrition-calculator ▾ Chipotle Mexican Grill ·
Chipotle Mexican Grill, USA, Canada and UK. Burritos, Tacos and more. Food With
Integrity

*Note: Some restaurants will only have nutrition facts and not a
calculator. This varies from website to website*

Step 3: Choose Your Meal

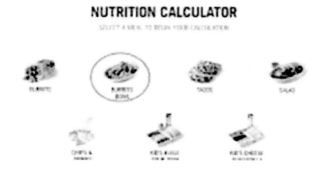

Step 4: Select Your Ingredients

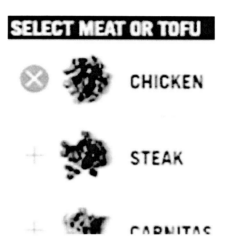

SELECT MEAT OR TOFU

⊗ CHICKEN

✛ STEAK

✛ CARNITAS

Step 5: Check the Nutrition Total: Calories and Macronutrients

TOTALS

SERVING SIZE (OZ)	18.5
CALORIES	650
CALORIES FROM FAT	210
TOTAL FAT (G)	22.5
SATURATED FAT (G)	11
TRANS FAT (G)	0
CHOLESTEROL (MG)	163
SODIUM (MG)	1380
CARBOHYDRATES (G)	61
DIETARY FIBER (G)	15
SUGAR (G)	4
PROTEIN (G)	44

Step 6: Create a New Food in MFP and fill in the details

6a)

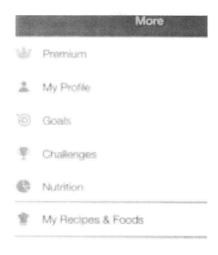

6b)

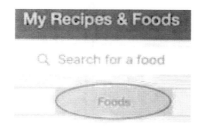

6c)

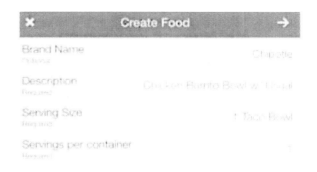

Step 7: Fill in Nutrition Info. (from Step 5)

7a)

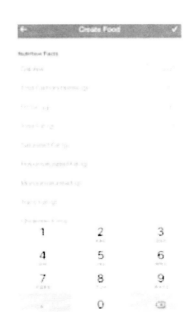

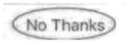

7b)

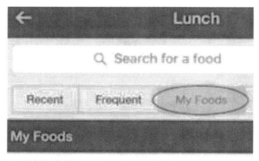

7c)

This is great, now I can add a chicken burrito bowl from Chipotle to any of my meals, whenever I choose to eat there again. Next time I eat out at Chipotle, I won't have to redo the process above! You can use this process with any restaurant meal you enjoy.

Unfortunately, not every restaurant provides easy-to-use online nutrition calculators like Chipotle's website. In most cases, they don't need to. You usually know what you're getting, and expecting, in most cases.

For example, In-N-Out Burger can easily be searched in MFP's database (use Method 1 from Ch. 3). I usually go with a "double-double burger". I search MFP for: *double double in n out*.

This method of eating out looks like this:

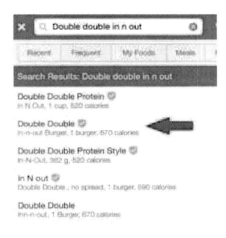

then

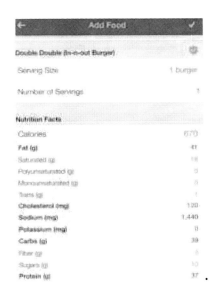

Not too bad right? If you felt like adding fries with that, you know what to do.

5.3 Eating Out (Nutrition Info. Unavailable)

There are times when restaurants don't provide nutrition information online or offline. This can be the case if you're in one of those, delicious "hole in the wall" type spots of town. Another occasion could be that you're at a more formal restaurant, eating at a social gathering, like a barbecue, or eating a hot dog at a ball game. Is there a way to log this in? Well, yes and no, we can use a rough estimate approach.

Let's use a traditional restaurant scenario; you've ordered a lean cut of steak and mashed potatoes. You noticed that the steak is 10 ounces according to the menu. The weight of mashed potatoes wasn't given. It's time to bring out MFP and search generic entries for both foods while you wait for the food to be served.

Lunch	595 cal
Steak Steaks, 10 ounce	475
Mashed Potatoes W/ Gravy Generic, 1 cup	120
+ Add Food	••• More

You can tailor this method to any scenario you encounter. Of course, it's not going to be 100% accurate, but "ballpark" will be good enough for these situations.

There's no reason to skip out on a restaurant meal because nutrition information wasn't available! Just do your best to stay within your caloric deficit, remember that's the key. Some flexible dieters don't log in foods, in such occasions, because it's not worth the hassle, for one, and two, because they know the food they're consuming won't push them over maintenance. Sure they're caloric deficit percentage won't be ideal, but they will not gain weight.

If you go overboard, it's not the end of the world. One day of over spillage won't kill you. However, if you make eating out a consistent habit, it might add up to very little visual progress, or worse, set you back for days.

As you can see, there's no silver bullet when it comes to eating out. There are different strategies for different scenarios at best. Being prepared with, at least, one of them makes it easier to gauge your intake and lessens the chances of gaining fat by making you aware of what you're consuming.

5.4 Moderation is Key

"If one oversteps the bounds of moderation, the greatest pleasures cease to please." – Epictetus

Everything in moderation. Will you never eat cookies or go out to a fast food join again? I doubt it; well, I know I couldn't at least. This is why I treat myself to these foods in moderation.

Moderation, in my experience, is having a maintenance day once a week. A day where I eat at equilibrium where I know I'm not going to be losing or gaining weight. The scale the next morning might rise, but I know it's temporary water weight, glycogen, and most importantly I know it's not weight from fat.

I usually have maintenance days on Fridays or Saturdays. Eating at maintenance once a week will not hinder your weight loss efforts. I believe their psychologically necessary actually, they're almost like reward days if you think about it.

Before I started IIFYM, I used to binge on fast foods. The scenario went like this: full>satisfied>bloated>uncomfortable>" wow why did I do that". And on some occasions, I drank alcohol on the same nights! This is a common combination that leads to fat gain.

It's worth noting that 1 gram of alcohol is equivalent to 7 calories.

When I go out to eat I stay within my daily macro budget. Going out to eat on a maintenance day is just a bonus. What other type of diet allows for this?! Rest assured, as long as it's not a daily habit, fast food is not off limits.

Action Step 4

Set up and save at least one of your favorite restaurant meals using any of the methods detailed in this chapter. Feel free to add in more meals. MFP will save your meal creations. Once saved you can access them at any time and them to your food diary.

Chapter 6

Tracking Your Progress

"Success is nothing more than a few disciplines, practiced every day."

– Jim Rohn

Body composition describes the percentage breakdown of the amount of muscle, body fat, bone and water our bodies are composed of.

You're going to want to be proactive by tracking numbers associated with your weight and waist circumference. You want to understand your body composition as much as possible throughout your fitness journey to always know if you're headed in the right direction.

In order to make sure you're on the right track, losing fat, not wasting time, and doing so in a healthy manner, measuring your progress is essential. In the words of Lord Kelvin, a physicist & engineer (who determined the correct value of a Kelvin (273°C)), "If you cannot measure it, you cannot control it". Measuring is a part of progressing and should be a weekly habit, and can even be a daily habit.

There are two main tools, outside of MFP, you're going to use to measure your progress and chances are you have these tools lying around somewhere.

6.1 *Weight and Pictures*

The weight scale is the iconic progress tracker when it comes to weight loss. Although it doesn't provide us with the whole story, on our progress, it's still useful.

Keep in mind that weight fluctuates depending on the time of day you weigh yourself. Throughout your journey, you might weigh yourself one day and seem to have lost a pound, and the next you're back at square one, or sometimes even a pound heavier. This is normal and is nothing to stress over. Everyone encounters this issue when they're in a caloric deficit, and you're not alone.

Many factors have an impact on weight fluctuations. A few of these factors are water retention, bowel movements, and glycogen storage. In order to get the most accurate scale reading we're going to measure by the weekly averages, not days. Weigh yourself at the same time every day. Make sure to do this first thing in the morning, on an empty stomach, as well as, after using the restroom to get the most accurate reading. At the end of every week take the average of your readings and note that it doesn't have to be every day of the week.

MFP can handle tracking your daily weight measurements.

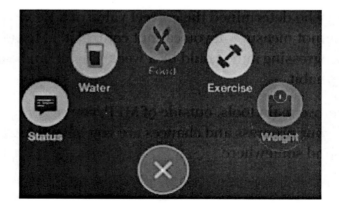

MFP also gives you the option to take photos, which I highly recommend, when you go to record your weight.

Pictures, along with mirror reflection analysis, will help you get a better understanding of how you're progressing. It's also really great to look back at your old photos and compare them with the new you! MFP lets you compare photos side by side, detailing both the date you took the picture and how much you weighed in that day.

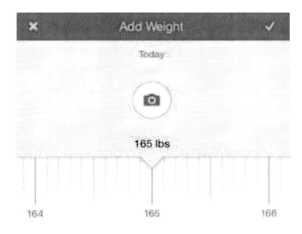

If you'd like to see your progress, at a glance, you can do so by selecting *Progress* in MFP's lower menu.

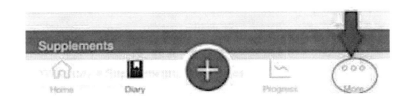

Selecting this will take you to a page where you can view the progress you've made. It allows you to view your past progress in a graph mode. The graph shows data points of your weight entries (the y-axis) and the date you recorded them (x-axis). You can also adjust the time frame of this graph by weeks, months, and years.

This is a handy feature that is much better than keeping a separate journal and having to manually record every day in my opinion. Be consistent and your graph will end up looking like a beautiful fluctuating mess (you'll see what I mean soon).

6.2 Waist

The second method of tracking progress is using a waist tape measure. A tape measure is arguably more revealing than the scale because you can potentially have a smaller weight on the same day the weight on the scale is stagnant. Along with photos, it can be a determining factor, to check, if you've truly gained weight or if your body is just retaining water. For those reasons, it's a good idea to measure your waist, just above the belly button, after you weigh in.

To get the most accurate reading, relax and don't suck in your tummy. Breathe as you normally would and get a reading.

MFP will track waist measurements in the same fashion it tracks weight.

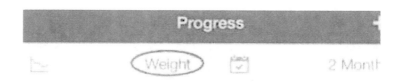

You can change the progress settings by switching "Weight" to "Waist" to record your waist measurement.

Select a Measurement

Weight

Neck

Waist

Hips

Conclusion

"It's your road and yours alone. Others may walk it with you, but no one can walk it for you." – Rumi

That's it; IIFYM mixed with a touch of today's technology. This approach to eating has allowed me to get my health back.

MFP is currently helping over 80 million users get closer and closer to their ideal body weight, many of whom follow IIFYM guidelines. I'd like to welcome you to the club!

My first goal with this book was to be a guide in a world where people are bombarded with the latest and greatest fad diets, magic pills, and food tracking naysayers. Nothing has, or ever will, trump the first law of thermodynamics, the law of energy balance. No so-called *fitness guru* can ever reverse one of the fundamental laws of the universe. My second goal was to create a resource for IIFYM that's not just informational, but applicable.

If you're new to If It Fits Your Macros, don't sweat it, take baby steps. Take the time to learn the lessons in this book and implement them as often as possible. You'll realize it's like riding a bike for the first time. Once you know how to do it you'll always know how.

The ultimate key to your success is to just to start. Start logging meals you eat into MFP, start weighing your foods, hitting your macros, start exercising and tracking your progress.

As the week's progress, you may notice that weight loss starts to get progressively tougher. It's nothing you can't handle! Weight loss is like any other goal. The goal gets tough towards the end stages. You see, our bodies want to hold onto as much fat as possible; it's how we're genetically coded. Picture your body as Gollum and your body fat stores as the One Ring (forgot to mention I'm a nerd at heart—Lord of the Rings reference). You're going to have to fight Gollum and his obstacles until you destroy your One Ring. Gollum is going to try to stump you every step of the way! The point is your body is smarter than you think, but knowing the power of energy balance, we can rest assure that the weight will continue to come off.

There will be obstacles on your road to success. It's inevitable. Success is never a crystal staircase. Most people think success is linear, but in fact it's quite messy! Take a look at a snapshot of my weight progress (via MFP). It's not pretty.

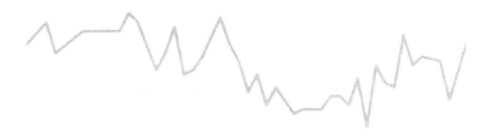

Allow yourself to make mistakes, but make sure to learn from them and never give up. Perhaps you'll make a few mistakes, such as overeating, or be tricked by scale fluctuations. These things will happen, but the important thing is to recover quickly and keep moving in the same direction as your goal.

If possible, make it a habit of combining: being in a caloric deficit and exercising (cardio and or strength training). This will only propel you to your goal faster.

Ralph Emerson once said "that which we persist in doing becomes easier – not that the nature of the task has changed, but our ability to do has increased" and his quote is extremely true when embarking on any goal. The good news is IIFYM is easy to be persistent in because the strict aspect of traditional dieting is absent.

A quick note, on the human body, the human body is a finely-tuned, piece of biological machinery and it will let go of fat when energy is demanded (a caloric deficit + exercise demands that your body digs into your fat stores for energy). I assure you the weight will come off in due time; your body will have no choice but to change if you follow the IIFYM principles outlined in this book.

IIFYM will separate you from the pack. Stop guessing like the rest of the world and get real, long lasting, results. When you start to see progress, that's the moment when you'll start loving the IIFYM approach.

Go after your fitness goals like there's no tomorrow—you're only here for a limited amount of time. I hope this book plays a role in getting you to the body and health you've always wanted.

CPSIA information can be obtained
at www.ICGtesting.com
Printed in the USA
LVOW10s1617200617
538750LV00012B/1086/P